Life After a Mental Health Diagnosis

CHAPTER 1: UNDERSTANDING YOUR DIAGNOSIS

- Exploring the specifics of your mental health condition, its symptoms, and its effects on your life.

CHAPTER 2: SEEKING SUPPORT

- Discussing the importance of finding a support system, including friends, family, therapists, support groups, and online communities.

CHAPTER 3: TREATMENT OPTIONS

- Exploring various treatment options such as therapy, medication, lifestyle changes, and alternative therapies.

CHAPTER 4: SELF-CARE STRATEGIES

- Offering practical tips and techniques for self-care, including managing stress, maintaining a healthy lifestyle, and coping with symptoms.

CHAPTER 5: BUILDING RESILIENCE

- Exploring ways to build resilience and adaptability in the face of mental health challenges.

CHAPTER 6: COMMUNICATING WITH OTHERS

- Discussing how to communicate effectively with loved ones, employers, and others about your mental health condition.

CHAPTER 7: NAVIGATING RELATIONSHIPS

- Addressing the impact of your diagnosis on relationships with family, friends, romantic partners, and coworkers.

CHAPTER 8: MANAGING WORK AND SCHOOL

- Providing guidance on managing your mental health while pursuing your education or career goals.

CHAPTER 9: OVERCOMING STIGMA

- Discussing the stigma surrounding mental health and strategies for combating stigma in your own life and in society.

CHAPTER 10: FINDING MEANING AND PURPOSE

- Exploring ways to find meaning, purpose, and fulfillment in your life despite mental health challenges.

CHAPTER 11: ADVOCACY AND ACTIVISM

- Discussing ways to advocate for yourself and others with mental health conditions, including participating in advocacy organizations and raising awareness.

CHAPTER 12: HOPE AND RECOVERY

- Highlighting stories of hope and recovery, and emphasizing that recovery is possible and achievable.

Introduction:

In the intricate tapestry of human experience, mental health plays a profound and often unseen role, shaping our thoughts, emotions, and interactions with the world around us. Yet, for too long, mental health has been shrouded in silence, stigma, and misunderstanding, leaving many individuals to navigate the complexities of their inner world alone.

This book, "Navigating Mental Health: A Guide to Understanding, Healing, and Thriving," seeks to illuminate the path toward greater understanding, compassion, and resilience in the face of mental health challenges. Drawing upon a wealth of knowledge, insights, and lived experiences, we embark on a journey of exploration, discovery, and empowerment, guided by the belief that every individual deserves to live a life of dignity, purpose, and fulfillment.

Through these pages, we will traverse the landscape of mental health, delving into the intricacies of diagnosis, treatment, and recovery with curiosity, empathy, and hope. From understanding the nuances of different mental health conditions to exploring strategies for self-care, advocacy, and finding meaning, this book offers a comprehensive roadmap for navigating the complexities of mental health with courage, resilience, and compassion.

Central to our exploration is the recognition that mental health is not a solitary journey but a shared human experience, woven into the fabric of our relationships, communities, and society. As we journey together, we will celebrate the stories of hope and resilience that illuminate the path toward healing and recovery, affirming that no matter how challenging the road may seem, there is always a glimmer of light to guide us forward.

It is our hope that this book will serve as a beacon of hope and empowerment for all those who are navigating the terrain of mental health, offering insights, tools, and support to help you navigate the challenges, embrace your strengths, and embark on a journey of healing, growth, and transformation. Together, let us embark on this journey of understanding, healing, and thriving, knowing that we are never alone in our quest for greater well-being and wholeness.

CHAPTER 1: UNDERSTANDING YOUR DIAGNOSIS

Exploring the specifics of your mental health condition, its symptoms, and its effects on your life.

Understanding your mental health diagnosis is the first step toward gaining insight into your condition and developing strategies for managing it effectively. In this chapter, we will delve into the complexities of various mental health conditions, shedding light on their symptoms and exploring how they may impact different aspects of your life.

Defining Your Diagnosis

Every individual's experience with mental health is unique, but diagnoses provide a framework for understanding and treating these conditions. Whether you've been diagnosed with depression, anxiety, bipolar disorder, schizophrenia, or another mental health condition, it's essential to gain a comprehensive understanding of what your diagnosis entails.

Symptoms and Manifestations

Symptoms vary widely depending on the specific condition, but common manifestations may include changes in mood, behavior, thoughts, or perceptions. Understanding the symptoms associated with your diagnosis can help you recognize when you're experiencing difficulties and seek appropriate support.

Impact on Daily Life

Mental health conditions can affect various aspects of your life, including relationships, work or school performance, physical health, and overall well-being. By acknowledging the ways in which your diagnosis influences your daily life, you can begin to develop coping strategies and make necessary adjustments to support your mental health.

Seeking Professional Guidance

Navigating a mental health diagnosis can be overwhelming, but you don't have to do it alone. Seeking guidance from mental health professionals, such as therapists, psychiatrists, or counselors, can provide invaluable support as you learn to manage your condition and improve your quality of life.

Embracing Self-Compassion

It's important to remember that having a mental health diagnosis does not define your worth as a person. Practicing self-compassion and cultivating a non-judgmental attitude toward yourself can help you cope with the challenges of living with a mental health condition and foster a sense of acceptance and resilience.

Conclusion

Understanding your mental health diagnosis is a crucial step toward empowerment and self-awareness. By familiarizing yourself with the specifics of your condition, recognizing its symptoms, and acknowledging its impact on your life, you can take proactive steps toward managing your mental health and achieving greater well-being.

In the chapters that follow, we will explore strategies for seeking support, managing symptoms, and navigating the journey of living with a mental health condition. Remember, you are not alone on this journey, and there is hope for healing and growth ahead.

CHAPTER 2: SEEKING SUPPORT

Discussing the importance of finding a support system, including friends, family, therapists, support groups, and online communities.

Seeking support is a crucial aspect of navigating life with a mental health condition. In this chapter, we will explore the significance of building a strong support system and discuss the various sources of support available to you.

The Importance of Support

Having a reliable support system can provide emotional validation, practical assistance, and a sense of belonging, all of which are essential for maintaining your mental health and well-being. Supportive relationships can help you cope with challenges, reduce feelings of isolation, and enhance your overall resilience.

Friends and Family

Friends and family members can play a significant role in supporting you through difficult times. By confiding in trusted loved ones and fostering open communication, you can cultivate meaningful connections that provide comfort, understanding, and encouragement.

Mental Health Professionals

Therapists, counselors, psychiatrists, and other mental health professionals can offer specialized support and guidance tailored to your individual needs. Seeking therapy can provide a safe space to explore your thoughts and emotions, learn coping strategies, and work toward healing and growth.

Support Groups

Support groups bring together individuals who share similar experiences and provide a forum for mutual support, validation, and learning. Whether in-person or online, participating in support groups can offer a sense of community, shared understanding, and valuable insights from others who have walked a similar path.

Online Communities

The internet has made it easier than ever to connect with others facing similar challenges. Online forums, social media groups, and virtual communities offer opportunities to share experiences, seek advice, and find solidarity with people from diverse backgrounds and perspectives.

Building Your Support Network

Building a support network may require reaching out to others, expressing your needs, and being proactive in seeking support. It's essential to identify individuals and resources that align with your values, preferences, and goals, and to prioritize self-care and boundaries in your relationships.

Conclusion

Seeking support is not a sign of weakness but a courageous acknowledgment of your own humanity and interdependence. By nurturing meaningful connections with friends, family, therapists, support groups, and online communities, you can cultivate a robust support system that empowers you to navigate life's challenges with resilience and grace.

In the chapters that follow, we will explore strategies for self-care, coping with symptoms, and fostering resilience in the face of adversity. Remember, you are not alone on this journey, and there is strength in reaching out for support when you need it most.

CHAPTER 3:
TREATMENT OPTIONS

Exploring various treatment options such as therapy, medication, lifestyle changes, and alternative therapies.

Navigating the landscape of treatment options is a crucial aspect of managing a mental health condition. In this chapter, we will explore a range of approaches to treatment, from conventional therapies to alternative modalities, empowering you to make informed decisions about your mental health care.

Therapy

Therapy, also known as counseling or psychotherapy, is a cornerstone of mental health treatment. Different modalities, such as cognitive-behavioral therapy (CBT), dialectical behavior therapy (DBT), psychodynamic therapy, and interpersonal therapy, offer diverse approaches to addressing symptoms, improving coping skills, and promoting emotional well-being.

Medication

Medication can be an effective tool for managing symptoms of certain mental health conditions, particularly when combined with therapy and lifestyle changes. Psychiatric medications, such as antidepressants, mood stabilizers, antipsychotics, and anti-anxiety medications, are prescribed by healthcare providers based on individual needs and treatment goals.

Lifestyle Changes

Making positive lifestyle changes can have a profound impact on mental health and overall well-being. Prioritizing sleep, nutrition, exercise, and stress management can enhance resilience, reduce symptoms, and support recovery from mental health challenges. Integrating mindfulness practices, relaxation techniques, and creative outlets into your daily routine can also promote emotional balance and inner peace.

Alternative Therapies

In addition to conventional treatments, many individuals explore alternative therapies to complement their mental health care. Alternative modalities, such as acupuncture, yoga, meditation, art therapy, and music therapy, offer holistic approaches to healing that address the mind, body, and spirit. While research on the effectiveness of these therapies varies, many people find them beneficial for reducing stress, improving mood, and enhancing overall quality of life.

Collaborative Care

Effective treatment often involves a collaborative approach, where healthcare providers work together to address the diverse needs of individuals with mental health conditions. Collaborative care models may include coordination between therapists, psychiatrists, primary care physicians, and other healthcare professionals to ensure comprehensive and integrated care.

Personalized Approach

There is no one-size-fits-all solution when it comes to mental health treatment. Each individual's journey is unique, and finding the right combination of therapies and interventions may require patience, experimentation, and ongoing communication with healthcare providers. By taking a personalized approach to treatment, you can tailor your care plan to suit your preferences, values, and goals.

Conclusion

Exploring treatment options is a proactive step toward enhancing your mental health and well-being. By considering a variety of approaches, from therapy and medication to lifestyle changes and alternative therapies, you can develop a comprehensive care plan that addresses your individual needs and supports your journey toward healing and recovery.

In the chapters that follow, we will delve deeper into strategies for self-care, coping with symptoms, and fostering resilience in the face of mental health challenges. Remember, you have the power to advocate for your own health and to seek out the support and resources that resonate with you on your path to wellness.

CHAPTER 4: SELF-CARE STRATEGIES

Offering practical tips and techniques for self-care, including managing stress, maintaining a healthy lifestyle, and coping with symptoms.

Self-care is an essential aspect of maintaining mental health and well-being. In this chapter, we will explore a variety of practical strategies and techniques to help you prioritize self-care and nurture your mind, body, and spirit.

Managing Stress

Stress is a natural part of life, but chronic stress can take a toll on your mental and physical health. Managing stress involves identifying sources of stress, developing coping strategies, and implementing relaxation techniques to promote a sense of calm and balance. Mindfulness meditation, deep breathing exercises, progressive muscle relaxation, and guided imagery are just a few techniques that can help you manage stress effectively.

Maintaining a Healthy Lifestyle

A healthy lifestyle forms the foundation of overall well-being. Eating a balanced diet, getting regular exercise, prioritizing sleep, and avoiding harmful substances such as alcohol and drugs can support mental health and resilience. Incorporating nutritious foods, engaging in physical activity you enjoy, and establishing a consistent sleep routine can boost mood, energy levels, and cognitive function.

Coping with Symptoms

Living with a mental health condition may involve coping with a range of symptoms, from mood swings and intrusive thoughts to panic attacks and sleep disturbances. Developing coping strategies tailored to your individual needs can help you navigate these challenges and maintain stability. Journaling, creative expression, practicing self-compassion, and seeking social support are valuable tools for coping with symptoms and promoting emotional well-being.

Setting Boundaries

Setting boundaries is essential for preserving your mental health and protecting your time, energy, and resources. Learning to say no to excessive demands, prioritizing your own needs, and communicating your boundaries assertively can reduce stress and prevent burnout. Setting aside time for self-care activities, establishing limits on work or social commitments, and seeking support when needed are crucial components of maintaining healthy boundaries.

Cultivating Positivity

Cultivating a positive mindset can enhance resilience and improve overall well-being. Practicing gratitude, engaging in activities that bring joy and fulfillment, and challenging negative thought patterns can shift your perspective and promote a sense of optimism. Surrounding yourself with supportive people, seeking out uplifting experiences, and focusing on strengths and accomplishments can foster a positive outlook on life.

Conclusion

Self-care is not selfish; it is a necessary investment in your own health and happiness. By prioritizing self-care and implementing practical strategies to manage stress, maintain a healthy lifestyle, cope with symptoms, set boundaries, and cultivate positivity, you can nurture your well-being and build resilience in the face of life's challenges.

In the chapters that follow, we will continue to explore ways to support your mental health journey, from fostering meaningful relationships to finding purpose and fulfillment in life. Remember, self-care is an ongoing practice, and small actions taken consistently can have a profound impact on your overall quality of life.

CHAPTER 5: BUILDING RESILIENCE

Exploring ways to build resilience and adaptability in the face of mental health challenges.

Resilience is the ability to bounce back from adversity, cope with stress, and thrive in the face of challenges. Building resilience is an essential skill for navigating the ups and downs of life, particularly when living with a mental health condition. In this chapter, we will explore strategies for cultivating resilience and fostering adaptability in the face of mental health challenges.

Understanding Resilience

Resilience is not a fixed trait but a dynamic process that can be developed and strengthened over time. It involves harnessing inner resources, coping skills, and support networks to overcome obstacles and persevere in the face of adversity. By cultivating resilience, you can enhance your ability to navigate life's challenges with courage, optimism, and determination.

Cultivating Self-Awareness

Self-awareness is a cornerstone of resilience, allowing you to recognize your strengths, limitations, and triggers. By cultivating self-awareness through practices such as mindfulness meditation, journaling, and reflection, you can gain insight into your thoughts, emotions, and behaviors, empowering you to respond to challenges with greater clarity and resilience.

Developing Coping Skills

Coping skills are tools and techniques that help you manage stress, regulate emotions, and cope with adversity. Building a toolbox of coping skills tailored to your individual needs can enhance your ability to navigate mental health challenges effectively. Techniques such as problem-solving, emotion regulation, and seeking social support can bolster resilience and promote emotional well-being.

Nurturing Support Networks

Social support is a powerful protective factor against the negative effects of stress and adversity. Cultivating strong relationships with friends, family members, support groups, and other sources of support can provide a sense of belonging, validation, and encouragement. By nurturing support networks, you can create a safety net of caring individuals who are there for you during difficult times.

Embracing Adaptability

Adaptability is the ability to adjust to changing circumstances and thrive in new environments. Embracing adaptability involves cultivating a growth mindset, embracing change as an opportunity for learning and growth, and being open to new experiences. By fostering adaptability, you can navigate life's twists and turns with resilience and flexibility.

Finding Meaning and Purpose

Finding meaning and purpose in life can provide a sense of direction, motivation, and resilience in the face of adversity. Engaging in activities that align with your values, passions, and interests, connecting with a sense of purpose larger than yourself, and seeking opportunities for growth and contribution can foster resilience and enhance overall well-being.

Conclusion

Building resilience is a journey that requires self-awareness, coping skills, social support, adaptability, and a sense of meaning and purpose. By cultivating these qualities and incorporating resilience-building practices into your daily life, you can strengthen your ability to cope with mental health challenges, navigate adversity, and thrive in the face of life's ups and downs.

In the chapters that follow, we will continue to explore strategies for supporting your mental health journey, from fostering meaningful relationships to advocating for your needs and rights. Remember, resilience is not about avoiding difficulties but about facing them with courage, resilience, and hope for a brighter tomorrow.

CHAPTER 6: COMMUNICATING WITH OTHERS

Discussing how to communicate effectively with loved ones, employers, and others about your mental health condition.

Effective communication is essential for fostering understanding, support, and collaboration when it comes to mental health. In this chapter, we will explore strategies for navigating conversations about your mental health with loved ones, employers, and others in your life.

Breaking the Silence

Opening up about your mental health can be challenging, but it is an important step toward seeking support and understanding. Breaking the silence surrounding mental health stigma involves challenging misconceptions, reducing shame and fear, and fostering open dialogue about mental health experiences.

Communicating with Loved Ones

Talking to loved ones about your mental health can be a source of comfort and validation. When communicating with family members, friends, or romantic partners, it's essential to approach the conversation with honesty, empathy, and vulnerability. Expressing your feelings, sharing information about your condition, and articulating your needs can foster understanding and strengthen your relationships.

Discussing Mental Health at Work

Navigating conversations about mental health in the workplace requires careful consideration of professional boundaries, confidentiality, and potential repercussions. When disclosing your mental health condition to employers or colleagues, it's important to assess the culture and policies of your workplace, communicate your needs and accommodations clearly, and advocate for support and accommodations as needed.

Seeking Support from Healthcare Providers

Effective communication with healthcare providers is crucial for receiving appropriate treatment and support for your mental health condition. Building a collaborative relationship with therapists, psychiatrists, and other mental health professionals involves sharing relevant information about your symptoms, treatment preferences, and goals, asking questions, and providing feedback on your progress.

Setting Boundaries and Asserting Your Needs

Assertive communication is essential for advocating for your needs and setting boundaries in relationships and interactions. Learning to assertively communicate your boundaries, express your needs, and negotiate compromises can empower you to navigate challenging situations and protect your mental health and well-being.

Educating Others and Advocating for Change

Beyond personal conversations, advocating for mental health awareness and education can help reduce stigma and promote understanding in your community and society at large. By sharing your story, participating in advocacy efforts, and promoting mental health resources and support networks, you can contribute to positive change and create a more supportive and inclusive environment for individuals with mental health conditions.

Conclusion

Effective communication is a powerful tool for fostering understanding, support, and connection when it comes to mental health. By approaching conversations about your mental health with honesty, empathy, and assertiveness, you can cultivate meaningful relationships, advocate for your needs, and contribute to a more compassionate and supportive society.

In the chapters that follow, we will continue to explore strategies for supporting your mental health journey, from managing relationships and navigating work environments to finding meaning and purpose in life. Remember, you are not alone, and there is strength in sharing your story and seeking support from others.

CHAPTER 7: NAVIGATING RELATIONSHIPS

Addressing the impact of your diagnosis on relationships with family, friends, romantic partners, and coworkers.

Living with a mental health condition can have a profound impact on your relationships with others. In this chapter, we will explore the challenges and opportunities that arise in navigating relationships with family, friends, romantic partners, and coworkers in the context of mental health.

Understanding the Impact

A mental health diagnosis can affect your relationships in various ways, including changes in communication patterns, emotional intimacy, and social interactions. Understanding the impact of your diagnosis on your relationships can help you navigate challenges and foster stronger, more supportive connections with others.

Communicating with Loved Ones

Open and honest communication is key to maintaining healthy relationships, especially when it comes to mental health. Talking to family members, friends, and romantic partners about your diagnosis, symptoms, and treatment can promote understanding, empathy, and mutual support. Sharing your feelings, expressing your needs, and setting boundaries can strengthen your relationships and enhance your well-being.

Managing Boundaries

Setting boundaries is essential for preserving your mental health and maintaining healthy relationships. Boundaries help clarify expectations, protect your emotional well-being, and promote mutual respect and understanding. Learning to assertively communicate your boundaries and negotiate compromises can help navigate challenging dynamics and promote harmony in your relationships.

Seeking Support from Loved Ones

Support from loved ones can be invaluable in coping with the challenges of living with a mental health condition. Whether it's emotional support, practical assistance, or simply being there to listen, having a supportive network of family and friends can provide comfort, validation, and encouragement during difficult times. Expressing gratitude, showing appreciation, and reciprocating support can strengthen your bonds and foster resilience in your relationships.

Navigating Romantic Relationships

Navigating romantic relationships can be particularly complex when one or both partners have a mental health condition. Open communication, mutual understanding, and empathy are essential for maintaining a healthy and supportive relationship. Discussing how your mental health affects the relationship, establishing boundaries, and seeking couples therapy or support groups can help address challenges and strengthen your connection with your partner.

Interacting with Coworkers

Navigating relationships with coworkers can present unique challenges in the workplace. While disclosing your mental health condition to colleagues is a personal decision, fostering open communication, setting boundaries, and advocating for accommodations can help create a supportive work environment.

Educating coworkers about mental health, promoting inclusivity, and seeking support from supervisors or human resources can contribute to a more understanding and supportive workplace culture.

Conclusion

Navigating relationships when living with a mental health condition requires empathy, communication, and mutual support. By fostering open and honest communication, setting boundaries, seeking support from loved ones, and advocating for your needs, you can navigate challenges and cultivate meaningful connections with family, friends, romantic partners, and coworkers.

In the chapters that follow, we will continue to explore strategies for supporting your mental health journey, from managing stress and coping with symptoms to finding meaning and purpose in life. Remember, you are not defined by your diagnosis, and you deserve love, understanding, and support from those around you.

CHAPTER 8: MANAGING WORK AND SCHOOL

Providing guidance on managing your mental health while pursuing your education or career goals.

Balancing the demands of work or school with the challenges of managing a mental health condition can be daunting. In this chapter, we will explore strategies for maintaining your mental health and well-being while pursuing your education or career goals.

Understanding Your Needs

Recognizing your unique strengths, limitations, and triggers is essential for effectively managing your mental health in work or school settings. Understanding how your mental health condition impacts your functioning, productivity, and well-being can help you identify strategies for managing stress, prioritizing self-care, and advocating for your needs.

Creating a Supportive Environment

Creating a supportive environment at work or school involves fostering open communication, setting boundaries, and seeking accommodations when necessary. Educating supervisors, teachers, or colleagues about your mental health condition, discussing potential accommodations, and advocating for supportive policies and practices can help create a more inclusive and understanding environment.

Managing Stress and Burnout

Managing stress and preventing burnout are crucial for maintaining your mental health in high-pressure work or school environments. Setting realistic goals, prioritizing tasks, and practicing time management can help reduce stress and improve productivity. Engaging in stress-reducing activities such as mindfulness meditation, physical exercise, and creative outlets can promote relaxation and emotional well-being.

Seeking Support and Resources

Seeking support from colleagues, classmates, supervisors, or teachers can provide valuable encouragement, validation, and assistance in navigating work or school challenges. Utilizing campus or workplace mental health resources, such as counseling services, support groups, or employee assistance programs, can offer additional support and guidance in managing your mental health.

Setting Boundaries and Self-Care

Setting boundaries and prioritizing self-care are essential for preserving your mental health and preventing burnout in work or school settings. Learning to assertively communicate your limits, delegate tasks, and take breaks when needed can help maintain a healthy work-life balance. Incorporating self-care practices such as regular exercise, adequate sleep, and enjoyable activities into your routine can promote resilience and well-being.

Advocating for Yourself

Advocating for your needs and rights in work or school environments is essential for ensuring access to accommodations, support, and opportunities for success. Communicating assertively, documenting accommodations, and seeking assistance from disability services or human resources can help address barriers and promote a more inclusive and supportive environment for individuals with mental health conditions.

Conclusion

Managing work or school while living with a mental health condition requires resilience, self-awareness, and proactive self-care. By understanding your needs, creating a supportive environment, managing stress and burnout, seeking support and resources, setting boundaries, and advocating for yourself, you can navigate work or school challenges effectively while prioritizing your mental health and well-being.

In the chapters that follow, we will continue to explore strategies for supporting your mental health journey, from fostering meaningful relationships to finding purpose and fulfillment in life. Remember, you are capable of achieving your goals while maintaining your mental health, and there is strength in seeking support and advocating for your needs along the way.

CHAPTER 9: OVERCOMING STIGMA

Discussing the stigma surrounding mental health and strategies for combating stigma in your own life and in society.

Stigma surrounding mental health remains a significant barrier to seeking support, receiving treatment, and living a fulfilling life for many individuals. In this chapter, we will explore the harmful effects of stigma, strategies for challenging stigma, and ways to promote acceptance and understanding in society.

Understanding Stigma

Stigma refers to negative attitudes, stereotypes, and discrimination directed toward individuals with mental health conditions. Stigma can manifest in various forms, including social exclusion, employment discrimination, and lack of access to healthcare. Internalized stigma, or self-stigma, occurs when individuals internalize negative beliefs about mental illness, leading to shame, self-doubt, and reluctance to seek help.

Examining the Impact

The impact of stigma on individuals with mental health conditions is profound and far-reaching. Stigma can exacerbate feelings of shame, isolation, and self-esteem, leading to delayed treatment, social withdrawal, and reduced quality of life. Stigma also contributes to disparities in healthcare access and outcomes, perpetuating cycles of discrimination and marginalization.

Challenging Stigma

Challenging stigma requires collective effort and action at multiple levels, from personal interactions to societal structures and policies. Strategies for challenging stigma include educating yourself and others about mental health, sharing personal stories and experiences, challenging stereotypes and misconceptions, and promoting empathy and understanding.

Promoting Open Dialogue

Promoting open dialogue about mental health is essential for reducing stigma and fostering understanding in society. Encouraging conversations about mental health, listening without judgment, and validating the experiences of individuals with mental health conditions can help break down barriers and promote acceptance. Creating safe spaces for discussion, such as support groups, educational forums, and community events, can provide opportunities for sharing stories, connecting with others, and challenging stigma.

Advocating for Change

Advocacy plays a crucial role in challenging stigma and promoting systemic change in society. Advocating for policy reforms, funding for mental health services, and anti-discrimination legislation can help address structural barriers and promote equal access to care. Participating in advocacy organizations, supporting mental health initiatives, and amplifying the voices of individuals with lived experience can contribute to positive change and social transformation.

Cultivating Compassion

Cultivating compassion and empathy toward individuals with mental health conditions is fundamental to combating stigma and fostering a more inclusive and supportive society. Recognizing the humanity and inherent worth of every individual, regardless of their mental health status, can help challenge stigma and promote acceptance. Engaging in acts of kindness, practicing active listening, and offering support and encouragement to those in need can create a culture of compassion and solidarity.

Conclusion

Overcoming stigma surrounding mental health is a collective responsibility that requires commitment, courage, and compassion from individuals, communities, and society as a whole. By challenging stereotypes, promoting open dialogue, advocating for change, and cultivating empathy and understanding, we can create a world where individuals with mental health conditions are valued, supported, and treated with dignity and respect.

In the chapters that follow, we will continue to explore strategies for supporting your mental health journey, from fostering resilience and managing relationships to finding meaning and purpose in life. Remember, your voice matters, and your actions have the power to make a difference in challenging stigma and promoting mental health equity for all.

CHAPTER 10: FINDING MEANING AND PURPOSE

Exploring ways to find meaning, purpose, and fulfillment in your life despite mental health challenges.

Living with a mental health condition can present unique challenges to finding meaning and purpose in life. However, it is possible to cultivate a sense of fulfillment and satisfaction by exploring activities, relationships, and pursuits that align with your values, passions, and aspirations. In this chapter, we will explore strategies for discovering meaning and purpose in the midst of mental health challenges.

Reflecting on Values and Passions

Exploring your values, passions, and interests can provide valuable insight into what gives your life meaning and purpose. Reflect on activities, relationships, and experiences that bring you joy, fulfillment, and a sense of accomplishment. Whether it's spending time with loved ones, pursuing creative outlets, or engaging in activities that align with your values, identifying what matters most to you can guide you toward a more meaningful life.

Setting Meaningful Goals

Setting meaningful goals can provide direction, motivation, and a sense of purpose in life. Whether it's pursuing educational or career aspirations, cultivating relationships, or making a positive impact in your community, setting goals that align with your values and aspirations can give your life meaning and direction. Break down your goals into manageable steps, celebrate your progress, and adapt your plans as needed to stay aligned with your vision for the future.

Cultivating Relationships and Connections

Relationships are fundamental to our sense of belonging, connection, and purpose in life. Cultivating meaningful relationships with family, friends, and community members can provide emotional support, validation, and a sense of belonging. Invest time and effort in nurturing relationships that uplift and inspire you, and seek out opportunities to connect with others who share your values and interests.

Making a Difference

Making a positive impact in the lives of others can give your life meaning and purpose beyond yourself. Whether it's volunteering for a cause you believe in, advocating for social justice, or supporting others in their journey toward recovery, finding ways to make a difference can bring fulfillment and a sense of meaning to your life. Look for opportunities to contribute your time, talents, and resources to causes that resonate with your values and passions.

Practicing Gratitude and Mindfulness

Practicing gratitude and mindfulness can help you cultivate a deeper appreciation for life's moments and experiences. Take time each day to reflect on the things you are grateful for, whether it's small moments of joy, acts of kindness from others, or the beauty of nature. Mindfulness practices, such as meditation, deep breathing, and sensory awareness, can help you stay present, grounded, and connected to the richness of life.

Embracing Personal Growth

Embracing personal growth and learning can enrich your life

and provide a sense of purpose and fulfillment. Be open to new experiences, challenges, and opportunities for learning and growth. Whether it's pursuing hobbies, acquiring new skills, or exploring new perspectives, embracing personal growth can help you expand your horizons, overcome obstacles, and discover new facets of yourself.

Conclusion

Finding meaning and purpose in life is a deeply personal and ongoing journey that evolves over time. By reflecting on your values, setting meaningful goals, cultivating relationships, making a difference, practicing gratitude and mindfulness, and embracing personal growth, you can discover a sense of fulfillment and satisfaction despite mental health challenges. Remember, your journey is unique, and there is no one right path to finding meaning and purpose. Trust in your own inner wisdom and intuition as you navigate the twists and turns of life, and embrace the opportunities for growth and transformation that come your way.

CHAPTER 11: ADVOCACY AND ACTIVISM

Discussing ways to advocate for yourself and others with mental health conditions, including participating in advocacy organizations and raising awareness.

Advocacy and activism are powerful tools for creating positive change and promoting the rights, dignity, and well-being of individuals with mental health conditions. In this chapter, we will explore strategies for advocating for yourself and others, participating in advocacy organizations, and raising awareness to reduce stigma and improve access to care.

Understanding Advocacy

Advocacy involves speaking up, taking action, and working to create systemic change on behalf of yourself or others. Advocacy can take many forms, from self-advocacy in personal interactions to broader activism aimed at influencing policies, practices, and public attitudes toward mental health.

Empowering Self-Advocacy

Self-advocacy is the process of speaking up for your own needs, rights, and preferences in personal and professional settings. Assertive communication, self-awareness, and knowledge of your rights and resources are essential for effective self-advocacy. Whether it's advocating for accommodations at work or school, seeking appropriate treatment and support, or challenging discrimination and stigma, empowering self-advocacy can help you navigate life with greater confidence and agency.

Participating in Advocacy Organizations

Joining advocacy organizations and support groups can provide opportunities to connect with others, share experiences, and amplify your voice on issues related to mental health. Whether it's local grassroots organizations, national advocacy groups, or online communities, participating in advocacy organizations can help you build solidarity, gain support, and effect change on a larger scale.

Raising Awareness

Raising awareness about mental health issues is essential for challenging stigma, promoting understanding, and fostering support in society. Whether it's sharing your story, participating in mental health awareness campaigns, or organizing events and activities in your community, raising awareness can help educate the public, reduce misconceptions, and encourage open dialogue about mental health.

Advocating for Policy Change

Advocating for policy change is a powerful way to address systemic barriers and promote equitable access to mental health care and resources. Whether it's advocating for increased funding for mental health services, supporting legislation to protect the rights of individuals with mental health conditions, or challenging discriminatory practices, engaging in policy advocacy can help create lasting change at the societal level.

Supporting Peer Advocacy

Supporting peer advocacy involves offering encouragement, validation, and assistance to others with mental health conditions in their advocacy efforts. Whether it's providing emotional support, sharing resources and information, or advocating alongside peers for common goals, supporting peer advocacy can strengthen solidarity and empower individuals to effect change together.

Conclusion

Advocacy and activism play a vital role in advancing the rights, dignity, and well-being of individuals with mental health conditions. By advocating for yourself and others, participating in advocacy organizations, raising awareness, and supporting policy change, you can contribute to a more inclusive, supportive, and compassionate society. Remember, your voice matters, and your actions have the power to make a difference in the lives of others. Together, we can work toward a world where mental health is valued, understood, and supported for all.

CHAPTER 12: HOPE AND RECOVERY

Highlighting stories of hope and recovery, and emphasizing that recovery is possible and achievable.

In the journey of mental health, hope shines as a guiding light, illuminating the path toward healing, resilience, and recovery. In this chapter, we will celebrate stories of hope and recovery, affirming that despite the challenges of living with a mental health condition, recovery is not only possible but also achievable.

Stories of Triumph

Throughout history and across cultures, individuals have overcome adversity and reclaimed their lives from the grip of mental illness. From artists and activists to athletes and everyday heroes, countless individuals have defied the odds, found strength in vulnerability, and emerged from darkness into the light of recovery. Their stories inspire us, reminding us that hope is a powerful force that can transform lives and shape destinies.

The Journey of Recovery

Recovery is not a linear path but a journey of growth, self-discovery, and resilience. It involves acknowledging the reality of your experiences, seeking support and treatment, and embracing the process of healing and transformation. Recovery is not about erasing the past or denying the challenges of mental illness; it's about reclaiming your sense of agency, purpose, and dignity in the face of adversity.

Finding Meaning in the Struggle

In the midst of struggle, there is often an opportunity for growth, meaning, and resilience. Many individuals with mental health conditions find that their experiences, though painful, have also shaped them into stronger, more compassionate, and more resilient individuals. Finding meaning in the struggle involves embracing the lessons learned, discovering inner strengths, and using adversity as a catalyst for personal growth and transformation.

Celebrating Milestones and Victories

Recovery is marked by moments of triumph, no matter how small or seemingly insignificant. From reaching out for help to taking the first steps toward treatment, every milestone along the journey of recovery is worth celebrating. Whether it's a day of stability, a moment of clarity, or a breakthrough in therapy, each victory reminds us that progress is possible and that hope is alive within us.

Nurturing Resilience and Self-Compassion

Nurturing resilience and self-compassion is essential for sustaining hope and resilience on the journey of recovery. Resilience involves cultivating inner strength, adaptability, and perseverance in the face of adversity. Self-compassion involves treating yourself with kindness, understanding, and acceptance, even in moments of struggle or setback. By nurturing resilience and self-compassion, you can weather life's storms with grace and resilience, knowing that you are worthy of love and belonging.

Supporting Others on the Journey

Supporting others on the journey of recovery involves offering empathy, validation, and encouragement to those facing mental health challenges. Whether it's lending a listening ear, sharing your own experiences, or providing practical support and resources, your presence and support can make a meaningful difference in someone's life. By offering hope and solidarity to others, you contribute to a culture of compassion and support where recovery is nurtured and celebrated.

Conclusion

Hope is not just a fleeting emotion but a powerful force that sustains us through the darkest of times and inspires us to reach for the light. In the stories of hope and recovery, we find inspiration, courage, and affirmation that no matter how difficult the journey may seem, recovery is possible and achievable. By embracing hope, celebrating victories, and supporting one another on the journey, we can create a world where everyone has the opportunity to thrive and flourish, despite the challenges of living with a mental health condition.

Conclusion:

As we come to the end of this journey through the intricacies of mental health, we are reminded of the resilience, courage, and compassion that reside within each of us. Throughout these pages, we have explored the depths of our inner landscapes, confronted the challenges of diagnosis and treatment, and celebrated the triumphs of recovery and healing.

In our exploration, we have encountered stories of hope and resilience, reminders that even in the darkest of times, there is light to be found. We have witnessed the power of empathy, connection, and support in nurturing healing and growth, affirming that no individual is ever truly alone on the journey toward greater well-being.

As we reflect on our experiences and insights, we are reminded that mental health is not a destination but a journey—a journey of self-discovery, growth, and transformation. It is a journey that requires courage to confront our vulnerabilities, resilience to overcome adversity, and compassion to extend to ourselves and others along the way.

As we close this chapter and step forward into the unknown, let us carry with us the lessons learned, the wisdom gained, and the hope ignited within our hearts. Let us continue to foster understanding, empathy, and acceptance in our communities and society, knowing that together, we can create a world where mental health is valued, supported, and celebrated.

May this book serve as a beacon of hope and empowerment for all those who are navigating the terrain of mental health, offering guidance, support, and solidarity on the journey toward healing, resilience, and thriving. And may we always remember that within the depths of our struggles lie the seeds of our strength, resilience, and infinite potential.

As we embark on the next chapter of our lives, let us do so with courage, compassion, and a steadfast belief in the power of hope and healing. For in the journey of mental health, there is always room for growth, connection, and possibility. Together, let us continue to navigate this journey with grace, resilience, and unwavering hope for a brighter tomorrow.